The Female Menopause Solution

The Female Menopause Solution

Taking care of your weight and hormones in the next phase of life

Dr. Beth Westie

This information is not intended or implied to be a substitute for professional medical advice, to diagnose, treat, cure or prevent any disease. All content is for general purposes only

ISBN: 978-0-9964457-5-7

Cover Design by Sianne Sprague
Formatted by Ann Aubitz – FuzionPress.com

First printing: 2019
23   22   21 20 19   5 4 3 2 1

Table of Contents

About the Author | 11

Part 1: Introduction to the Big Fat Problem | 14

Chapter 1: The 140-Pound Man | 19
Kathy | 19
Gender Differences in Males and Females | 20
Women Lose weight differently than men | 21

Part 2: Understanding Your Cycle | 23

Chapter 2: How Your Hormone Cycle Works in
Menopause | 25
How to Track Where You're At | 25

Chapter 3: Perimenopause | 28
Symptoms of Perimenopause | 28
More on Symptoms | 30

Chapter 4: Menopause | 35
Helen | 35
Symptoms of Menopause | 36
More on Symptoms | 37

Chapter 5: The Estrogen Phase | 41
The Cooling Phase – Foods to Focus On | 41
Other Ways to Enhance

the Cooling Properties of Estrogen | 42

Carbs and Estrogen | 42

Exercise during the estrogen phase | 42

Chapter 6: The Progesterone Phase | 45

The Warming Phase – Foods to Focus On | 45

Other Ways to Enhance the Warming

Properties of Progesterone | 46

Carbs and Progesterone | 46

Fasting/Cleanse Day | 47

Exercise during the progesterone phase | 47

Chapter 7: Planning Nutrition Cycles—

Failing to Plan is Planning to Fail | 49

Robin | 49

Part 3: Nutrition Basics for Women | 53

Anne | 54

Chapter 8: How Nutrient Recommendations

Change in Menopause | 57

Protein | 58

Plant vs. Animal Proteins | 59

Carbohydrates | 60

Fats | 60

Chapter 9: Nutrition Fundamentals | 63

Shelly | 63

Going Gluten Free | 64

The Dairy Dilemma | 64

Eat more leafy green veggies daily | 65

Benefits of Eating Organic | 65

Limit Sugar and Salt | 65

Avoid Over-processed Foods | 65

Read the Label | 65

Protein Increases | 66

Stay Hydrated | 66

Watch Portion Sizes, a.k.a., Portion Distortion | 66

Protein Pacing | 66

Nutrition and Mindset | 66

Beet Root | 67

Wine | 67

**Part 4: Exercise Basics for Women in Perimenopause
and Menopause** | 67

Barbara | 69

Chapter 10: Getting Started—Overall Approach to

Exercise | 70

Exercise strategies: | 73

Resistance/weight training | 73

Interval training | 74

Exercise and cortisol | 74

Chapter 11: Exercise and mindset | 75

Chapter 12: Detoxing for Women in Menopause | 77

Part 5: Other Important Factors That Impact Results | 79

Chapter 13: Mindset | 81

Mindset Tactics | 81

Chapter 14: Time it Takes for Things to Change in

Menopause | 83
Connie | 83

Chapter 15: Visceral Fat and Inflammation | 87

Chapter 16: Sleep | 89
Routines for sleep | 89

Chapter 17: Stress and Cortisol | 91

Chapter 18: Getting back on track: You fell off the wagon, now what? | 93

Chapter 19: Value of Herbs and Supplements to Your Overall Health | 95

Chapter 20: Hormone replacement | 97

Part 6: In Conclusion | 99

Praise from those who successfully used Dr. Westie's program | 101

Resources | 107

Acknowledgments

I want to express my sincerest gratitude to those who have supported me on this journey. I would not be where I am without your support. I am so grateful for the hundreds of women who have trusted me to guide them on their health journey, I am forever grateful. I am able to continue living my passion to the fullest because of you! This book is dedicated to giving women the answers they deserve in this phase of life!

About the Author

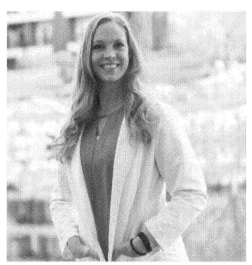

Doctor Beth Westie was born and raised on a small goat farm in Eagan Minnesota. After collecting a pair of state volleyball titles as an Eagan Wildcat, her sights turned to higher education in the form of The NMU Wildcat.

Being the recipient of a full athletic and academic scholarship to Northern Michigan University, Dr. Westie was able to combine her love of sport alongside her passion for women's health.

Upon graduating NMU with a bachelor's in biology and physiology, Dr. Beth Westie enrolled in the chiropractic program at Minnesota's Northwestern Health Sciences University. From there she went on to open and run a highly successful chiropractic office where she treated many women with hormone dysfunction and was able to help alleviate and resolve conditions ranging from infertility, weight gain, and inability to lose weight and keep it off, menstrual cycle issues, menopause, and more. It wasn't until then, that her passion for women's health and wellness could awaken and transform the lives of women around the world. After selling her highly successful Chiropractic practice, Dr. Westie jumped full time into speaking, and coaching.

Dr. Westie is the author of The Female Fat Solution, an Amazon Best Seller and #1 New Release. She is also the host of The Female Health Solution Podcast.

In the last couple years Dr. Westie has spent her time traveling the country, educating women and working to revolutionize the future of women's health. Appearing on local news stations in Minnesota, Colorado, North Dakota, Virginia, Illinois, and Vermont. Dr. Westie has dedicated her life to changing the way women look at their health, and lose weight through speaking, online programs, and private coaching.

She lives in Minnesota with her husband, son, and two daughters.

How to get the most out of this book

The Female Menopause Solution was written as a continuation of The Female Fat Solution book. There are core teachings and methods that are outlined in The Female Fat Solution will give you a more in depth explanation of information. I know you are busy, so I chose to make the Female Menopause Solution more concise by not repeating the same information from the first book.

If you're like me, and want a done-for-you program that fits specifically for your body, you'll want to get on the waitlist for the next 12 Week Program. In these programs, you will receive more specific guidance on how this works for you, based on your health history, hormone history, goals, dietary restrictions and more. Getting on the waitlist will give you a sneak peek at what working together looks like, and how to get started improving your health—now!

Get on the waitlist at www.drbethwestie.com/waitlist

Part 1

Introduction to the Big Fat Problem

*O*ne morning, I woke up with a tire around my waist that I hadn't asked for. Accompanying that tire were hot flashes, insomnia, and a body that felt like it belonged to someone else. I had been healthy all of my life. I maintained a healthy diet and exercised, yet no matter what I tried, the weight just kept coming. I had heard plenty of menopause horror stories, but I was determined that wasn't going to be me, so I did what worked in the past — counting calories and exercising more. That used to work when I wanted to drop some weight quickly. Now — nothing.

During a visit to my doctor, I was told my options were hormone replacement or cleaning up my diet. I felt dismissed. Like hello, I feel that I have no control over my body. Surely, there has to be something more to this. I went home and did what any women struggling would do — I went to Google. I was getting more of the same. Cut calories, lower carbs, exercise more. I've tried all that. I just knew there had to be something more.

When I came across Dr. Beth, I felt like she was speaking directly to me. I'm not going to lie, I had no idea I still had a hormone cycle. But knowing this information and that I could use it to figure things out gave me hope. I began following her suggestions, and low and behold, a few months in, the tire was shrinking, I was sleeping better, my energy was back and I felt in control again. Not only control, but I finally felt like I wasn't going to have to struggle any longer, because I knew my body.

You're probably feeling a little lost, which is why you've picked up this book. Maybe you woke up with what seems to be a tire that you didn't ask for around your midsection, and hot flashes that show up at the worst possible time. You've likely done nothing different, and you might even be doing all the "right things." Yet you are still struggling, and no one seems to have answers. You've likely been dismissed by your doctor, and told to exercise more or cut calories. I'm also guessing you've tried the things that used to work to lose weight, and they aren't working anymore. And let's not even get into sleep, or lack thereof.

The resources for women in menopause are slim. No one is researching it, and no one is talking about it. Women are left to struggle while media markets to women that hot flashes are normal. All of this can make women feel crazy. Things change and shift in their bodies, and they are left feeling that it's typical to feel like crap.

News flash: These symptoms may be common, but they **aren't normal**. Neither is the struggle that seems to be just a stage you have to get through at this point of life.

I'm here to tell you this isn't true.

You aren't supposed to struggle through menopause, sweating with the window open in the middle of winter, dealing with insomnia and weight gain. You aren't supposed to just exercise more to lose the weight that seems to have crept on overnight. The advice you are being given is BS. There are things you can do nutritionally to support your body through this phase so that you can thrive, and not just survive. And you definitely aren't supposed to feel bad about what's going on.

There is so much more that goes into deciphering your body in this phase of life. If it were as easy as a math equation (calories in minus calories out) we'd likely all have the body we want.

I'm also here to tell you that you aren't alone.

I get hundreds of messages each week from women who are frustrated and struggling with their menopausal body, unsure of where to turn next, and feeling like they're lost in the forest without the right map.

The Menopause Solution is that map. It's meant to serve as a guiding light to help you better understand that what you are going through is common, and you can turn things around. It is meant to give you the tools you need to better understand your body, start feeling good again, and lose the weight.

Chapter 1

The 140-Pound Man

Kathy

Kathy was healthy, active 55-year-old woman who had been fit her entire life. She knew what to do when she felt like she wanted to lose a couple pounds or tone up a bit. As a busy, working woman, she never struggled with her weight or her energy until she reached menopause.

"I had been in shape my entire life," she said. *"I was active, ate well and just never struggled. When I started going through the change, it felt like I had completely lost control of my body. All of my tried-and-true tricks to help me lose weight weren't working anymore. My husband suggested we go on this popular diet together, and I agreed.*

It wasn't long before I was even more frustrated than before we began. He was still drinking beer and eating pizza while seemingly shedding pounds by the minute, and here I was following this plan to a T with zero results.

I just could not understand what was going on. It was frustrating, to say the least. When I found Dr. Beth, I was at a really low point. I had been struggling with Menopause, my weight, and my energy for a couple of years now.

Everything she said made so much sense to me, and I knew she was the person I needed to work with to get things back on track.

I wanted more than a weight loss program. I wanted to truly understand what my body was doing and why, so that I never ended up in this place again. That's exactly what I got. I learned more about my body in the 12 weeks with her than I had over the course of my entire life.

My energy is back up, I feel like I finally have control of my body again, and I've officially lost the tire around my waist! I could not be more grateful to have found Dr. Beth when I did."

How could this happen? Women have been treated the same as men in terms of health and nutrition for a very long time, with no regard to the hormonal changes that they have not just throughout the month, but their entire lifetime! The ONLY changes that women are told to make nutritionally throughout their life is when they are pregnant. When a woman goes through menopause, her body is going through lot of hormonal changes. During this time, nutrition and fitness routines need to change to match that hormonal shift.

There is no research—I repeat, NO research—done on women and nutritional needs in the menopausal space. Therefore, women are following all these recommendations from research and data collected on men, with NO regard to the nutritional changes that women need.

Gender Differences in Males and Females

Men are from Mars, women are from Venus. The male body can more easily build muscle and drop body fat percentage. Women—especially when going through menopause—store fat more easily, and stress or hormonal changes kicks that fat storing up a notch or two! At the same time, it becomes more difficult to build and maintain lean muscle! So it's no wonder you feel like the cards are stacked against you. I also want to mention with weight and energy changes/issues, there is often an underlying feeling that there is a core health problem. Those changes are normalized for women, however, leading them to feel crazy for believing there's an underlying issue, thus igniting a sense of worry.

Women have been practically killing themselves for years trying to achieve the same results as their male counterparts, all the while following a plan not designed to work for them.

Women lose weight differently than men!

The female body is created differently than the male body, and it changes throughout our lives. Therefore, we gain and lose weight differently than men! If you are looking for lasting success with weight loss, the order of success looks different than what you've been told.

When on the correct plan for their bodies, women should begin to have more energy and better sleep, while noticing you are getting hungrier. Second, you will lose inches, and this drop in size often comes in a top-down fashion. Arms, chest and bust will get smaller, followed by the waist, hips and thighs. After these changes, the number on the scale can change, and your weight can have a lasting change. The purpose of this order will not just change the scale, but your body composition will also change, a result you get to keep! It is vital that women in menopause have these changes in the correct order—too often, we will try to cut calories and end up feeling depleted and lacking energy. This directly leads to quitting the plan you started, and feeling defeated that you can't do it. In reality, it's not your fault!

Women are constantly searching for the one "thing" that will help them FINALLY achieve and maintain the result they are looking for, but there is almost no information out there. We are the ones that are searching for it! Women who look for advice about their bodies are really reading and finding things that are for men. *Example of all athletic performance products are tested on 18 to 22-year-old male division one college athletes. And so many women who are looking to get the next-level results are using these same products, in the same way, and end up frustrated as to why it doesn't "work" for them!

It's also important to remember that it's not one thing that's going to be the be-all, end-all for results—no one diet, restriction, supplement or training session. It's a combination of things that work, because you have a new body now. You must eat for your new body to become and stay healthy.

Part 2

Understanding Your Hormone Cycle

Chapter 2

How Your Hormone Cycle Works in Menopause

How to track where you are at

In Perimenopause, you may have irregular periods, but can still track based off the most recent cycle that you had. In menopause, even though the hormones are decreased, they are not completely nonexistent. Some health professionals compare the menopausal body to be more similar to a man's body, hormonally. I disagree with this comparison, as it has not been on the same hormonal journey that the menopausal woman has been on.

It's also important to note that your body will continuously go through that hormone cycle, it's just on a smaller scale. There is a lot of benefit in following nutrition for your cycle and layering in seed cycling to enhance the effect of the remaining hormones (levels).

Often, women are told, "You don't have any hormones anymore, so it doesn't matter," but many women start following a hormone nutritional pattern and have a very positive reaction.

Keep in mind that these hormones go everywhere in the body, affect all other systems and cross the blood brain barrier, so they are very important.

If you're looking for an easy place to get started with nutrition that matches your cycle, head to my website www.drbethwestie.com/resources to get your free copy of my Recipes for Your Cycle Cookbook. It's full of healthy, easy-to-make, delicious recipes that help balance hormones naturally.

Chapter 3

Perimenopause

True perimenopause is the gradual/eventual decrease of progesterone and estrogen. Hormones that are high when you ovulate (LH and FSH) then elevate, and remain elevated for the rest of your lifetime. Often, a blood or saliva test is used to diagnose. There are some symptoms of perimenopause (and menopause) such as mood swings, fatigue, decrease in focus, irregular periods and hot flashes that can look like other things (such as thyroid or more serious diseases—I don't want this to be a scary fact, but I feel it's important to note). Usually, women put up with symptoms for long periods of time because they attribute the issues to something else.

Perimenopause is a difficult time for women, and unfortunately, not a lot is known about this stage. It's often overlooked, and for any symptoms that they may be struggling with, women are just told to "wait it out." It can be very difficult to navigate, as your experience may be completely different than your mother's or sister's.

Overall, it can take one to 10 years to fully move through the peri-stage. It's similar to getting your cycle to regulate at the start of puberty (which can take two to six years, but most people don't give it that amount of time and try to intervene with birth control) only in reverse. That means if it takes three years to get a cycle regular to start when a girl reaches puberty, the beginning of the process, the same time frame can be used going through perimenopause, the end of the process. It can take three years to completely go through this phase.

Factors that can affect the duration and symptoms of perimenopause include overall health, toxicity (exposure internal or external), history of illnesses, stress and more.

This can also be an emotionally difficult stage, as they body starts to change in ways you've never experienced or expected, and you cannot control all of it.

It is difficult to predict body's reactions to regular activities and stressors as hormones fluctuate up and down. Many of the "symptoms" or issues women experience shift with their health routine, but the result of any change is not immediate. Just like if we start a "diet" on a Monday, we can't expect to get to our goal by Wednesday that same week. If a positive health change is implemented, it may take weeks or even months to fully see the results of that change, which can be frustrating and difficult to track!

Symptoms of Perimenopause

What are some symptoms? Symptoms can include, but not limited to: Regular or irregular periods (What? it can be both? Yep—it's almost like this is the "no rules" phase that you have to go through) hot flashes, breast tenderness (all month long, or worse than you've had previously with PMS), worse PMS (any previous symptoms you experienced the week before your period can be amplified), decreased libido, vaginal dryness, night sweats, fatigue, weight gain, inability to lose weight, memory difficulties, depression and/or anxiety, urinary changes (having to go more frequently or having leakage), mood changes, sleep issues (insomnia like issues). All of these symptoms tend to start out of nowhere when women aren't doing anything different, which can be really tough.

Why are these symptoms happening? This is the menopause transition phase— when hormone levels are shifting and changing, and they do this in their own time and pattern. It is different for every woman and can have a different overall duration. Average timeline for perimenopause (menopause is defined as a full year, 12 months, without a menstrual cycle) is four years. But it can last for as little as one year, or up to a decade.

Natural methods of handling the shifting hormones are eating for your cycle—increasing protein and other nutrients to match the body's changing needs—and incorporating seed cycling (the process of using different seeds in one's diet at different times of the hormone cycle to help support hormone regulation). Managing stress and sleep will also improve overall symptoms through perimenopause.

More on Symptoms

Hot flashes: Hot flashes can be very disruptive occurrences for women. They can come on anytime, anywhere, stopping you in your tracks. The irregular nature of them is frustrating, because you can't predict them. They can last for 10 seconds to 10 minutes. You can have one a week, or one an hour! (That may be a bit of an exaggeration, but when you're having them, it can feel that way.) Hot flashes are prompted by hormone drop, and your body attempting to regulate and navigate around it. When waking at night from hot flashes, adrenaline can also increase, making it difficult to calm the body and mind enough to fall asleep again.

Adrenals and stress: DHEA drops affect how your body processes cortisol, playing a role in the negative effect of stress on the body, as well as weight gain and inability to lose weight, a continued response to negative stress in the body. If you are at a stage of adrenal fatigue when entering this stage of life, it will make the entire transition that much tougher. A big hill to climb as you are trying to navigate through this difficult phase.

Headaches: As with big shifts in hormones changing irregularly (hot flashes, irregular period), stress response difference, sleep, etc., can bring on terrible headaches, or even migraines throughout this stage.

Heart palpitations: These can be noticed as a result of imbalance of parasympathetic and sympathetic nervous systems—be sure to seek out your doctor if they increase in frequency and duration (but also don't be surprised or feel like a freak of nature for having them).

Heavy periods: A drop of progesterone and higher estrogen can cause more buildup in uterine lining, causing heavier than normal periods. Higher body fat (fat produces estrogen!) also can lead to having heavier periods.

Sleep disturbances: As your hormone levels drop, specifically estrogen, it decreases the body's ability to get into and stay in deep sleep (REM sleep). It can be tougher to fall asleep, and you wake more in the middle of the night.

Weight gain/Inability to lose weight: Estrogen is responsible for metabolic boosts regularly, so the drop in estrogen makes it easy for the body to shift to even more fat storing, especially around your abdomen and midsection—the tire you carry around your waist. Estrogen also helps with insulin sensitivity, but as estrogen levels drop, it's easy to become insulin-resistant, which means your body produces more insulin and triggers the storage of more nutrients as fat (great!). This blood sugar level up-and-down can affect your moods, focus, hunger and overall energy levels. DHEA (dehydroepiandrosterone, produced by your adrenals and ovaries) drops. DHEA is in charge of neutralizing cortisol's effect, and it does this by allowing your system to use stored glucose as energy. Without it, it's easier to become more sensitive to glucose and store as more belly fat/add to the tire around your waist. As it drops, it can be tougher to recover from episodes of stress and trauma (overwork, mental stress, physical stress, temperature changes, etc.).

Muscle breakdown: The rate of protein breakdown is higher, so it can be more difficult to build/synthesize and maintain lean muscle for strength and body composition. Studies have shown (ROAR, page 42) that women of perimenopause and menopause burned 23 to 33 percent less fat during exercise than women of younger ages.

Gut issues. Bloating and digestive changes can occur during this time. Because hormones can fluctuate a lot during perimenopause, it can contribute to a wide range of digestive issues. You can go from being constipated to having diarrhea, then be bloated and gassy. Your body will start to change how it processes sugars, salts and more. This also plays a role in energy and fluid retention.

Energy and fitness. Your energy may begin to fluctuate at this point. The shift in hormone affects the ups and downs of energy, and this may be exhibited in the fitness arena. Some workouts may feel powerful and some may feel exhausting, even if it's the same workout done just a week apart. Body temperature regulation during this time can also be difficult, as the hormones are changing.

Chapter 4:

Menopause

Helen

Helen was a recent empty nester who lived a busy life. Between work and life functions, she was always on the go. Helen struggled with her weight for almost her entire life. Recently, hormone and autoimmune issues added to her struggles.

"My weight had been a struggle for my entire life, or as long as I can remember," she said. "Basically, I had always yo-yo dieted, jumping from one thing to the next, hoping it was going to be the answer.

As I got older, it seemed like it became harder and harder to lose the weight. I hit menopause, and then it seemed like things spun out of control.

When I started working with Dr. Beth, it was so refreshing to find someone that looked at me as a whole. We talked about my hormone issues, autoimmune issues, and my struggles with weight loss. She set up a plan specifically for me to address all of these things at once.

It was life-changing—the best investment I've made in my health. I had no idea I could feel this good. I am confident the tools I have been given have set me up for the rest of my life.

My menopause symptoms are gone, autoimmune issues are under control, and I'm down 27 pounds and 30 inches overall. I feel like I have my life back."

Menopause is technically classified as a female not having a menstrual cycle for a full year, and can be determined by blood tests and measuring LH and FSH (luteinizing hormone and follicle stimulating hormone) levels high. Some women arrive at this stage, their period stops, and they don't notice any intense symptoms of being menopausal. Other women notice every little change their body makes throughout this period of time, and when menopause finally arrives, they want to be relieved—but that doesn't mean that their symptoms stop. At this point, women have a totally new body.

Symptoms of Menopause

Menopause is officially having no cycle for 12 months, so many of the perimenopausal issues won't be present here. Overall changes that are present (and here to stay) are thinner skin, more difficulty building lean muscle and maintaining lean muscle mass, increased tendency to store fat (increased body fat percentage even with continued healthy habits) insomnia/difficulty sleeping, energy levels, muscle building ability, change in libido, vaginal dryness, mood change, bone loss, skin changes, and potentially more.

Why are the symptoms happening? The main cause of these symptoms is that the ovaries stop producing estrogen, the hormone mainly responsible for these things.

More on Symptoms

Hot flashes: Once a woman has reached the end of menopause, her hot flashes should subside, but some women experience hot flashes for years afterward (so don't feel crazy if this is YOU!), Just know there are some great nutritional tweaks you can make to reduce the hot flashes in this stage. For most women, the hot flashes subside and it's a welcomed change!

Adrenals and stress: DHEA has dropped, affecting how the body processes cortisol. This plays a role in the negative effect of stress on the body, and also weight gain and inability to lose weight, a response to a continued increase of negative stress in the body). If you have had a lot of unmanaged stress in your life up until this point, it makes it more difficult to escape the negative impact of stress and inflammation on the menopausal body. The healthier you were, the more you can manage. Certain amounts of stress are still necessary to create and build strength, but it's not to be overdone.

Headaches: Even though the large shifts in hormones are done fluctuating, some women continue to experience headaches on a monthly basis, though often not as bad/severe as they were in the perimenopause stage.

Heart palpitations: If you experienced these during perimenopause, they should have subsided once in full menopause.

Sleep disturbances: Sleep can still be more difficult at this time. With lower hormone levels, falling asleep and staying asleep is sometimes a challenge.

Weight gain/inability to lose weight: Estrogen is responsible for metabolism boost regularly, so the drop in estrogen makes it easy for the body to shift to even more fat storing, especially around your abdomen and midsection-the tire you carry around your waist. Estrogen also helps with insulin sensitivity, but as it drops it's easy to become insulin resistant. This means your body produces more insulin, and triggers the storage of more nutrients as fat (great!). This blood sugar level up-and-down can affect your moods, focus, hunger and overall energy levels. DHEA dehydroepiandrosterone, produced by your adrenals and ovaries) drops. DHEA is in charge of neutralizing cortisol's effect, and it does this by allowing your system to use stored glucose as energy. Without it, it's easier to become more sensitive to glucose and store more belly fat/add to the tire around your waist. As it drops, it can be tougher to recover from episodes of stress and trauma (overwork, mental stress, physical stress, temperature changes, etc.).

At this point, women often become very frustrated with their inability to lose weight and lack of progress. Most women continue to try many different things to achieve results, and often, the tactics they are using are actually more damaging to the metabolism than helpful. This pattern can continue for years, leading to decreased muscle mass and increased fatty tissue.

Muscle breakdown: During this time, the rate of protein breakdown is higher, so it can be more difficult to build/synthesize and maintain lean muscle for strength and body composition. Studies have shown (ROAR, page 42) that women of perimenopause and menopause burned 23 to 33 percent less fat during exercise than women of younger ages. The rate of muscle breakdown can continue as it was in perimenopause stage, leaving women with decreased energy and decreased physical strength. Changes in nutrition and exercise focus can maintain, and even slowly increase, lean muscle tissue in the body.

Gut issues: Bloating and digestive changes may now feel like they are permanent. The digestive issues women have— constipation, bloat and gas—are going to feel more regular. It is important that nutrient-dense foods are eaten, as the digestive system doesn't absorb the necessary elements from food like it used to. The body now processes sugars and salts differently, so a careful look at the balance of carbohydrates is essential. The change in nutrient absorption also effects energy and fluid retention.

Energy and fitness: Energy may have reached a settling point now. As hormone levels are now stagnant, energy may feel tough to maintain, but can be positively impacted by daily nutrition and movement.

Chapter 5

The Estrogen Phase

During the estrogen phase, you may notice increased energy, better digestion, muscle building, carb burning, faster recovery from workouts and more mental focus.

The Cooling Phase: Foods to Focus On

During this phase, it's very beneficial to focus on cooling foods, which bring cool and calm energy to the body and can help increase natural carb-burning function. Foods such as turkey, fish, chicken, raw fruits and vegetables, as well as cool drinks and limiting caffeine are beneficial during this phase.

We can also emphasize the function of this phase using seasonings and herbs that match with estrogen.

Some warming tactics can be very helpful for digestive issues, and used on a regular basis. To offset the warming component, it is helpful to override it with more cooling properties.

Other Ways to Enhance the Cooling Properties of Estrogen

- Meditations
- Wearing cooling colors
- Cold showers
- Ice packs
- Skin care (aloe, coconut oil with peppermint oil)
- Essential oils (peppermint, spearmint, eucalyptus, bergamot, lemongrass, lime, vetiver)
- Avoid exposure to toxic chemicals
- Seed cycling (Pumpkin seed and flax seed; 1 tablespoon of each, raw and ground. Add to salads, smoothies, protein balls, etc., each day of the first two weeks, days 1-14.)
- Spices: basil, mint, sage, fennel, dill, parsley, rosemary

Carbs and Estrogen

Carbohydrate balance: The body processes carbs and sugars differently (more sensitive to carbs, more blood sugar fluctuations and craving carbs, but less need for carbs.) Moderate the carb amounts, and follow carb cycling patterns to keep metabolism going.

Exercise during the Estrogen Phase

During the estrogen phase, you'll want to focus on power and strength for training, and not so much on endurance. It can take longer to warm up and work up a sweat, so dress in layers to help warm up quicker, protecting muscle tissue, ligaments and joints from injury.

Post workout recovery is important, in order to help muscle tissue rebuild and decrease the stress response naturally. More on this later.

Chapter 6

The Progesterone Phase

During this phase, you may notice decreased energy, slowed digestion, longer recovery from exercise, and an overall higher body temperature. It's important to monitor core body temperature during workouts, as vasodilation – blood vessels increase in diameter allowing an increase in blood flow- decreases. That means it is more difficult to get to your sweating point and warm up, as well as cool body down, so easier to get overheated.

The Warming Phase: Foods to Focus on

Warming foods are very beneficial to focus on during the progesterone phase. They bring heat and energy to the body and can help increase natural digestive processes, as well as help increase core body temperature and blood flow. Some examples include beef, bacon, red meats, cooked fruits and vegetables, coffee and hot tea (caffeine).

Other Ways to Enhance the Warming Properties of Progesterone

- Seed cycling: Sesame seed and sunflower seed, 1 tablespoon of each, raw and ground. May be added to salads, smoothies, protein balls and more. Eat each day of the last two weeks, days 15 to 28.
- Spices: cinnamon, ginger, nutmeg, cayenne
- Hot showers
- Heating blanket
- Physical heat
- Essential oils: myrrh, juniper, black pepper, cardamom, cinnamon, clove, hyssop

Carbs and Progesterone

Carbs must be balanced during this phase, as they are essential in properly providing energy to the cells. Carb glucose gives energy to each cell, and your brain uses glucose as energy. Carbs are also helpful for fat metabolism (having the energy from carbohydrate to have a healthy metabolism that can burn more fat).

Other things to remember:

- Endurance training can be more difficult to attain—it's tougher to get to an endurance increase standpoint.
- Keep the main thing the main thing—don't get distracted by trendy things.
- Get solid nutrition and focus on movement. Results from your efforts are going to take much longer to flourish physically, but don't get discouraged. First changes that women normally notice (when following better nutrition and exercise for their hormones) are an increase in natural energy, better mental focus, improved sleep, and increased overall feeling of wellbeing.

Following a decreased carbohydrate diet (in attempt to reach ketosis to tap into fat-burning stores) often backfires for women in this stage. It can take much longer for the female in menopause to reach ketosis on a keto or similar-type diet, and can often trigger weight gain, making the scale creep higher than it already has.

Fasting/Cleanse Day

Intermittent fasting is a great way to temporarily enter a ketosis state safely for women, as long as it's done in a supported fashion. Going without nutrients for an extended period of time is counterintuitive. I recommend that women add in small, specific snacks to fasting days to avoid putting the body into fat-storage mode.

There are many patterns of fasting: 16/8 (16 hours fasting, 8 hours feeding), 5/2 (5 days of normal eating, and 2 days of fasting), and 24-hour. But keep in mind, many of these patterns and data on the benefits are focused on men. Women following these patterns will usually have short-term positive results, but long-term negative results.

Exercise during the Progesterone Phase

It can take longer to warm up and begin sweating, so dress in layers to help warm up quicker to protect muscle tissue, ligaments and joints from injury. On the flip side, it can be more challenging to cool down during and after exercise, as the body doesn't cool from sweating as much anymore. Be sure to monitor your core body temperature and track any signs of overheating.

Chapter 7

Failing to Plan Nutrition Cycles is Planning to Fail

Robin

"Menopause hit me like a ton of bricks. Hot flashes, night sweats, insomnia, weight gain…you name it, I had it. It seemed like everywhere I turned there were only Band-Aids to put over these things—no real fixes. I tried hormone replacement and it seemed like it made things worse.

I tried to dig in and research, and asked friends, doctors, and my mom. No one had a real answer for me except 'This is just part of this phase of life.'

When I found Dr. Beth, it was like finally someone was speaking my language. I knew I didn't want to struggle through this, and she was the only real person that gave me hope. I joined her program and was astonished. There was so much I didn't know about my body it was almost embarrassing.

Learning that my body was still having a hormone cycle even after a hysterectomy blew my mind. But when I started adding cooling and warming foods, it was like my body was thanking me for finally doing something right. My symptoms started to subside, I felt better, my energy was back, and it was incredible.

The things I learned in this program will serve me for the rest of my life. I've told every woman I know about Dr. Beth because I truly feel she saved me from years of struggle and frustration."

In overall planning, it's key that protein pacing is applied on a regular basis. All the salad in the world is not going to give you the energy that protein pacing will. Plan your day, week and month to crush your nutrition goals. Get to the grocery store while keeping in mind that you won't be going through the same buying routine as you did before. Your nutrition should be different to match what your system needs. Be sure to create your grocery list based on what your focus foods are for that phase. Start out by filling your cart with fresh fruits and vegetables, and lean proteins. Limit buying things that come in a box!

Plan for more protein. Your body needs more in menopause, as it doesn't upload the same as it did before. It takes more protein to do the same job as it did before. If you're eating the same—even if it's super healthy—you're missing the basic nutrient your body needs.

This is also a time to realize that most areas of your life are changing or going to change. Your health needs are different—not worse, necessarily—than they were before, so planning differently to match will make things a lot easier! Your exercise needs are different as well, and planning out these different routines, including a little more strength training, can go a long way in getting better results. If you're unsure of how or what to do, this is a perfect time to hire a trainer to help assist you in the new direction you are going.

Self-care is also going to be crucial to include in a daily routine—including stretching for flexibility, seeing a chiropractor regularly to maintain mobility, and adding massage therapy for muscle tension. Include other healthy routines like yoga, strength training, walking, meditation and other new activities.

Your relationships with a significant other and close friends may also change. These changes are easier to navigate with some reflection and planning on what you would like from the relationship going forward. As your body changes, don't be surprised with other changes with yourself. And as with any relationship, if one factor changes, it can alter the dynamic of the relationship. This doesn't have to be a bad thing, but experiencing dynamic changes within yourself and not anticipate it to affect close relationships may leave you unprepared.

As with any big hormonal change, it is normal to shift your lifestyle to accommodate—as with pregnancy, you change your eating habit and exercise habits, and with this major shift in hormones it is time to do the same.

Part 3

Nutrition Basics for Women in Menopause

Anne

"It's no secret that things change as we age, but I never truly thought it would be so tough to find answers. For my entire life, I had things mostly under control. I would diet here and there, I always felt like I could lose a bit of weight.

When I hit menopause, it was like I woke up one morning with a layer of fat over my muscle and a tire around my waist that was not moving, no matter how much I begged it to.

On top of that, sleep became an issue. Never in my life (okay, aside from when I had babies) did I struggle like this with sleep.

I searched and searched, but could not find a solid answer that made me feel like there was hope. I honestly thought I would just have to struggle through this phase, and hopefully, come out the other side.

A friend sent me a video Dr. Beth had done on how the body processes nutrients differently in menopause, and I was blown away. She was speaking about me. It felt like she had been spying on me. I was that person who hadn't really changed anything, but was gaining weight in what felt like the blink of an eye. I was doing NOTHING differently.

Did you know that the body processes carbohydrate differently in menopause? Or that it takes more protein to do the same job? Yeah, me neither.

I'm a smart woman, but all of this was new to me. When I joined Dr. Beth's program, I was desperate to end the madness. I didn't want to keep gaining weight, and I wanted my sleep back. Most of all, I wanted my life back.

Truth be told, as I was gaining this weight I wasn't able to do the things I loved anymore. I would get tired so fast, and not have the energy or the motivation.

I can honestly say that 12 weeks later, I am a completely different person. The value I drew from this program was unlike anything I had ever experienced. Don't get me wrong, I was skeptical at first. Would this really be the thing to work for me? What if I fail again? How can I spend this money on me?

I would do it 100 times over. I'm down 16 pounds and over 20 inches, my clothes are fitting again, my energy is back and my sleep has improved. I cannot say enough about this."

Chapter 8

How Nutrient Recommendations Change in Menopause

Keep in mind that these nutritional changes are meant to be integrated with any other positive nutrition changes that work for you—for example, if you are already gluten-free or paleo. This way of eating is a perfect synergy to an already healthy diet! Because of digestive system and energy-use changes with perimenopause and menopause, nutrient recommendations also change. You can still enjoy your favorite foods and eat at your favorite restaurants, but perhaps change the frequency and amount of those dishes to meet the new needs your body has.

It is often recommended that women entering and already in menopause increase their digestive breakdown and motility ability, and those components slow with aging. Adding a high-quality extra probiotic in the morning and a digestive enzyme at the largest meal of the day can help greatly with the digestive process. This will assist in the breakdown of nutrients, such as protein, to make sure you are absorbing the maximum amount possible from the food you eat. The most important thing to keep in mind is to eat nutrient-dense food, as empty calories that don't hold any value for you are now more harmful than ever.

Protein

You will need more protein on a daily basis. Protein pacing is a great way to take in more protein over time, rather than suddenly overloading your system with one large, high-protein meal. Protein pacing means consuming moderate amounts of protein at regular intervals throughout the day. This allows the body to upload that protein in even levels, and not overwhelm the digestive system.

The following is a protein pacing example (keep in mind this is **an example**, your protein amounts should be customized for you).

Protein Pacing Example
Breakfast: Meal with 20 grams of protein
Snack: 20 grams of protein
Lunch: Meal with 20 grams of protein
Snack: 20 grams of protein
Dinner: Meal with 20 grams of protein
Total = 100 grams for the day

The key to protein pacing is ensuring consumption is spaced out, about three hours apart for max digestion and upload, while achieving a higher total for the day. An important note to keep in mind is that your total protein pacing number will be specific to you, and can change with goals or activity or stress. For example, I am 6'2" and an athlete, busy mom and entrepreneur. I get about 180g of protein each day to stay energized and maintain enough muscle mass to perform at my peak!

If you're looking for easy, delicious ways to add extra protein to your diet, head to my website www.drbethwestie.com/resources for a copy of my High Protein & Fat Bomb Recipe Book. It's full of recipes like donuts, bars, muffins, ice cream and more! All packed with protein, delicious and healthy!

Plant vs. animal proteins: This topic is controversial, as there are many opinions of what types of proteins people should eat. My goal is to educate you on the options so you can make the best decision for yourself. Eating a mainly plant protein diet has a lot of health benefits, and it can be easier on the digestive system. But be wary of products that claim they are vegan or vegetarian, but use cheap fillers in the products— these are actually harder on your gut. It also can be more difficult to get the full spectrum of amino acids in only plant- based sources.

It's essential to consume a wide variety of beans, seeds, nuts and legumes for all the essential and nonessential amino acids. Animal proteins (especially cow-based beef and dairy) have the full spectrum of amino acids in them, making it easier and faster to help build lean muscle and burn more fat (in fact, some studies that show that grass- fed beef helps do both simultaneously). The downfall, of course, is to make sure you have clean sources—organic and grass-fed is best. Side note—if you have cut out animal protein for a period of time and want to try incorporating it back in your diet, your body will not have the enzymes to digest it, so slowly incorporate animal protein back into your diet to allow your system to acclimate.

Carbohydrates: Carbohydrates are processed differently in this stage. It is important to have a balance of simple and complex carbs, but you may not need as many carbs per day as you did before.

Simple carbs include things like sugar and fruits. Examples of complex carbs are potatoes, rice, pasta and breads. The body can become more sensitive to carbs, and it may be easier to experience blood sugar swings—this can be balanced with higher protein and fat levels in combination with the carbs. Included are alcohol sugars! I know, it's sad that drinking the same amount of wine can contribute to weight gain and inability to lose weight. But it does pay off to monitor alcohol consumption, and if you do have a glass, be sure to pair it with healthy fats and protein (a fat bomb and protein ball) to keep blood sugars more level.

Fats: Essential fatty acids, also called healthy fats, are necessary because your body can't produce these nutrients on its own. At this point, healthy fats are essential to maintain nutrient levels and support healthy hormone production. Healthy fat intake can be slightly higher to help maintain blood sugar levels daily. This can be one of the toughest nutrients to get in because of the old mindset of "fat will make you fat," and old fad diets that centered on little to no fat. Many women have to get over the mindset that eating fat consistently would be bad.

Micronutrients (Vitamins and minerals): As the digestive process slows, it can be more difficult to get in the essential micronutrients you need. Be sure to consume foods that are nutrient-dense (spinach, kale, avocado, blueberries, salmon, and more) to keep nutrient levels high. It is easy to overeat but be undernourished, if you are consuming lots of food that is processed and doesn't contain valuable nutrients. Adding a high-quality multivitamin or beverages that are boosted in vitamins and minerals can also be helpful, as long as they are not too high in sugar. Be cautious that the beverages you add don't have any artificial ingredients in them (like Gatorade). I like Nuun, as it has electrolytes and is a clean product.

Chapter 9

Nutrition Fundamentals

Shelly

"When I looked back, I realized I was slowly gaining weight for a really long time. It was never a lot all at once. It just slowly crept up, and I really didn't do a whole lot about it.

It wasn't until my son proposed to his girlfriend that I started to panic. I quickly realized there would be events to attend, and pictures taken. My confidence hit an all-time low, and I knew I needed to do something quickly.

I tried a few things that had worked when I was younger—counting calories, exercise and cleaning up my diet, but my weight was not budging.

A coworker of mine had been losing some weight, and overall just looked amazing. When I asked her what she was doing, she referred me to Dr. Beth.

I had never heard anyone talk about women's bodies and hormones the way Dr. Beth did. It made so much sense, and I quickly realized the things I was trying were likely making the situation worse.

When I reached out to her with my goal of losing a decent amount of weight, she was confident that I could get there. It was refreshing to hear someone lay out what the next three to six months of work would look like in terms of how my body would respond.

It felt like I knew exactly what to expect, and I was patient, because I kept the final outcome in mind.

Rather quickly, I started to realize how deep of a hole I was in. When I started gaining energy I didn't ever realized I had lost, I was confident we were on the right track. It took some time, but my body started changing. Losing inches and seeing the shift was amazing.

I'm happy to say I showed up to my son's wedding looking and feeling my best, and I am so grateful!

The following are some nutritional guidelines that you will find helpful as you plan your nutrition and right diet for your body.

Going gluten free: Cutting gluten and some grains can be very helpful to decrease the inflammation in the digestive system, which can aid in increasing nutrient absorptions and decrease bloat.

The dairy dilemma: Decreasing or cutting dairy can be a tough decision. On one hand, dairy can be a great source of protein, especially when protein pacing and consuming high-protein snacks. Dairy can also be inflammatory and increase mucus production, contributing to bloating and digestive discomfort. To help increase protein daily using dairy, try adding in a digestive enzyme to help decrease bloat if you have it with dairy.

Eat more leafy green veggies daily: The increase in fiber in leafy greens can be beneficial for the digestive system, as well as the vitamins and minerals. The greens should be cooked slightly for optimal absorption. Steaming or lightly sautéing more fibrous vegetables helps with digestive process. Some of my favorite leafy greens are spinach, kale and chard.

Benefits of eating organic: Eating organic means the food contains more nutrients than conventionally grown foods, and don't have chemicals (that can be endocrine disruptors).

Limit sugar and salt: Sugar and salt are often added to processed foods to add flavor, but this adds to damaging blood sugars and weight gain. Avoiding processed foods as much as possible can significantly cut down on unnecessarily added sugars and salts

Avoid over-processed foods: There are negative impacts when consuming artificial flavors and colors, along with the sugar and salt intake that accompany over-processed foods.

Read the label: Check the protein-to-carb ratio of the foods you're consuming to ensure higher protein-to-carb amounts throughout the day—this will help with protein pacing and moderating carb intake. Add sugars up throughout the day to track amounts—it's useful to track the nutrients you're getting each day by using an app.

Protein increase: In menopause, it takes more protein to create the same effect it used to, with the decrease of muscle tissue (women experience a decrease in energy, and feel flabbier as their muscle decreases and fat tissue increases). To combat this, increase your protein intake.

Stay hydrated: Drink water and mineral-boosted water throughout the day to ensure full hydration uploading into the cells. I like to alternate a bottle of water with a bottle of electrolyte drink all day.

Watch portion sizes: Because nutrient needs are different in this phase of life, the portions on your plate will look different than before. Ensure higher protein amounts and lower carb amounts, with more leafy greens.

Protein pacing: Increase protein intake to add nutrients to fuel muscle tissue growth and maintenance. Protein pace each meal and snack.

Nutrition and mindset: You have a new body, new hormone levels, new nutritional needs and you will need a new mindset to go with it. It doesn't have to be a bad thing that your hormones are not at the same level they used to be. It just means you can have a different mindset about how your body functions. This will allow you to have an easier time transitioning to your new body.

Beet Root: Add beet root to help increase oxygen levels in the body—throughout menopause, it can be harder.

Wine: With research listing some health benefits, I had to include a section on wine. A few things to keep in mind when looking at your wine intake: wine adds empty calories, can worsen hot flashes, is harder on your liver (and your liver is doing enough right now) and thus, it can be something that's holding you back. Try cutting it out for at least 30 days to see how you feel!

Part 4

Exercise Basics for Women in Perimenopause and Menopause

Barbara

"My weight was affecting a lot more than just my self-confidence. The turning point for me was when I began looking at some of my health markers and knew things were trending in the wrong direction.

I was only 55. I wanted to be around to not only see my grandkids grow up, but also to be an active part of their lives. My husband and I had always been super active, but as my weight crept up, that activity level plummeted. I knew if I didn't do something, things were only going to get worse.

I had stumbled upon Dr. Beth's podcast, and when I reached out to her I was nervous. I've tried a lot of different weight loss plans, and spent more money than I care to admit. I was terrified that this would be another one of those things that I tried and failed. Reassurance came when I understood how this program would be adjusted to fit me, and how my body was responding. No one had ever done that before for me.

I knew it was the right fit. The communication and customization I got from Dr. Beth was incredible. Any concern I had she addressed immediately, and was more than willing to help adjust things as I needed.

I can happily say that I am down 31 inches overall, but what I am more proud of is my health markers finally going in the right direction. My energy is back, and I am able to actually play with my grandkids.

My husband told me the other day how proud he was of me for taking control of my health and doing something for me. I am so grateful to Dr. Beth for guiding me through this, and helping me get my life back.

Chapter 10

Getting Started: Overall Approach to Exercise

New exercise strategies will mean changing up your routine to achieve the best results with growing and maintaining lean muscle, which improves body composition quickly.

Exercise Strategies

Resistance/weight training: Focus on weight lifting for more muscle growth and maintenance. It's more difficult to gain and maintain muscle tissue, and weight lifting is key to combating this. Not just any weight lifting, but focusing on power during the training sessions is key. The best way to achieve this is to increase weight amount and do fewer reps. Then, do three to four sets. Example: typical set of lunges, if you usually do two sets of 15 holding 10-pound weights in each hand, the next level up is doing three sets of eight reps holding 20-pound weights.

Nutrition timing around these workouts is also key to ensure the max muscle building and recovery. The new (menopausal) body has a more difficult time building and maintaining muscle after workouts. The goal of workouts is to breakdown the muscle fibers to rebuild it stronger and denser. Without proper protein and BCAA post-workout, the body doesn't get to rebuild the muscle, and recovery is not attained. Muscle recovery is the muscle fibers repairing as quickly as possible post-workout, and healing the damage.

Interval training: Cardiovascular health is still important, and can be maintained by interval training. Long gone are the days of spending hours on the treadmill to keep in shape. Interval training is more efficient and produces faster results. An example is burst training, such as tabata: 20 seconds of higher intensity followed by 10 seconds of low intensity (example—20 seconds of running, and then 10 seconds of walking). The length of rest can also be increased if needed, as you are getting in better shape for this type of training.

Exercise and cortisol: Cortisol should be carefully monitored, as it can hamper the results you are trying to achieve. The menopausal body is more sensitive to recovering from cortisol, so it's essential that you train within the proper timing for nutrition, as well as duration. Fasted workouts should be avoided, and any exercise longer than 45 minutes should have a snack break built in. Other stress in life can be managed well with meditations, adaptogens, and deep breathing patterns. Increases in cortisol can decrease the recovery rate from exercise.

Chapter 11
Exercise and Mindset

For women in perimenopause and menopause, changing the type, frequency, and intensity of exercise can provide a much better result. Although shifting exercise can improve body composition, it may not be the type of exercise you are used to or enjoy. Find a way to integrate this into your routine in a fun way. It is most helpful to find a group of other women to workout with to keep the routine enjoyable.

Also, the changes to mindset can be a different journey. As hormones shift and change through perimenopause and menopause, it can cause mood changes. Hormones cross the blood brain barrier, so it is normal to have changes of mindset and mood during this time. Finding a routine that is fun is key. Joy is now higher on the priority list!

Chapter 12
Detoxing for Women in Menopause

Detoxification is essential for everyone, but especially for women in perimenopause and menopause. Just living in our current world, we are exposed to many toxins, and our bodies are not designed to process the type and quantity of these toxins, both externally and internally. Therefore, some type of detoxification is necessary. It's also important to note that this is typically the first step I recommend when working with women. If you are trying to lose weight and haven't flushed out excess hormones in the body, it's comparable to being on a sinking ship that has 10 holes, and only patching one. You aren't going to get the result you truly desire.

Detoxification can be done in many ways, but often it is best to start slowly, especially if you haven't done a detox before. The type of detox is important. Doing an intestinal detox can help with any digestive issues, but the more lasting and impactful detox is a liver detox. Yes, your liver is designed to detox your body, but the sheer amount of crap your body must filter through is too much for the modern liver to handle. That, combined with year and years of environmental and internal stress, old injuries, scar tissue, inflammation, illnesses, etc., it's too much for your little liver to handle. Assisting the liver with its regular detoxification helps achieve a new level of results, and maintain them. It's important to note that a liver detox is something I recommend women have some guidance on. This is not going to look the same for everyone, and should be custom to your body and where you're at.

If you're ready for a specific protocol you, you'll want to get on the waitlist for the next 12 Week Program. This is the first step, during which we address and customize for each individual so that they're starting off on the right foot.

Go to my website and get on the waitlist so that you're the first to know about the next group: www.drbestwestie.com/waitlist.

Part 5

Other Important Factors that Impact Results

Chapter 13

Mindset

Addressing mindset is really important, especially when going through a big transition like menopause. You have a completely new body in this phase of life, and it's important to understand that just because things are different, it doesn't have to be negative. If you set appropriate expectations for your new body, you will be less likely to feel frustrated. Getting used to your new body and different expectations doesn't mean that the old thoughts and expectations just go away. Set new ones, and as they start influencing new ways to think, feel, and act, the old expectations begin to fade. Give yourself the time to shift, and you will achieve and stay the positive outcomes.

Mindset Tactics

Set realistic goals. Set goals based on where your current starting point is, and make sure you have a plan in place that can help get you there.

Do not compare. Your body is completely different than what it was before menopause, so it's unfair to compare the two. Give yourself some grace.

Focus on the positive. Find the things that are positive in your life at the moment. Whatever you focus on, you are going to get more of, so it might as well be good!

Find gratitude. Take five minutes each day to write down three things you are grateful for. When you continue to focus on what you have instead of what you don't, you will feel more overall satisfaction.

Celebrate your wins. We can get so caught up in a number. It's important to celebrate all of the small victories on the way to your big goal.

When it comes to mindset, it's also important to understand how you have developed that mindset around nutrition. Most likely it came from your environment. If your mom or dad cooked things a certain way, you likely cook in a similar fashion. Growing up, if you were taught certain foods were good or bad, you ma y still have the same thoughts.

If you were like me, you watched other female adults in your life go through fads with nutrition that helped shape how you view foods. Maybe it was buying all low-fat products, or swapping margarine for butter. Whatever it may have been, it probably left an impact—and maybe not a positive one.

If you're ready to take a good look into where your mindset about nutrition is at and what you may be able to improve on, visit my website at www.drbestwestie.com/resources, and download your free copy of my Food Habit Blueprint. It's a great exercise to take an in-depth look at how your nutrition mindset has been programmed.

Chapter 14

Time it Takes for Things to Change in Menopause

Connie

" I was diagnosed with a thyroid condition years ago, but it seemed like just recently, things began to spiral out of control.

I was struggling with fatigue, weakness, weight gain, depression, and so much more. It felt like I was on a rollercoaster ride trying to figure it out what to do.

I really didn't find help anywhere. My thyroid numbers were in the normal range, so the solution I was given was to eat less and workout more, but I knew there had to be more to it than this, and it was frustrating. Struggling without answers is something I wouldn't wish on my worst enemy!

A friend of mine who had also been struggling with similar issues sent me a YouTube video by Dr. Beth, and it was like a lightbulb went on. I binge-watched her videos for hours. I had never heard anyone talk about women's health and hormones in that way. Things were finally making sense to me, and I knew she was the woman I wanted to talk to.

When I explained what I was going through, she made me feel heard. I could tell she understood and actually cared to help me. Working with her for 12 weeks was the best decision I had ever made.

I know that if I hadn't taken that step, I would still be spinning my wheels, trying to put the pieces together myself.

I can't even explain how quickly I started feeling better. The fatigue is gone, my sleep is back to normal, and I've finally started losing weight again. I know I will be able to continue on with this for the rest of my life."

The time and effort required to obtain visible physical changes can feel like it takes a lot longer in menopause. The female body can build more muscle (pre-menopause) when estrogen is higher in days 1 to 14 of the cycle, so when estrogen levels drop, it's more difficult to build muscle and see changes. At most, the female body will build half a pound to one pound of lean muscle a week with optimal power training and nutrition (pre-menopause), so after hormone levels change and drop—specifically estrogen—muscle tissue growth is much more difficult to achieve, and therefore will take longer.

Typically, a woman who achieves visible results in 8 to 12 before menopause can expect post-menopausal to take 16 to 20 weeks to notice results. It's important that women note these timeline changes, as it is very easy to get discouraged when trying to work out and eat right with a specific result in mind. One of the most frustrating things women experience with weight gain in menopause is that it seems like the weight just creeps on overnight, yet doesn't come off. For women of menopausal age to see results, expect to change training and nutrition tactics and consistently apply them for a minimum of 12 weeks to start to notice the changes.

The difficult thing for women to get behind is that these changes begin on the inside, and don't provide any external measurement of results that match the amount and time of effort. You have to shift your mindset, and should be prepared to endure a longer time. You have to set a new timeline on the calendar to take markers and data points.

When first implementing dietary changes, the initial results (loss of inches) may appear from eliminating processed foods and immediately decreasing the inflammation in the body, but these results are not part of the body changing in muscle and fat tissue composition. They are exciting to experience, but not part of any lasting changes for the physique.

Changes often appear in patterns for women. A noted increase in energy and better sleep, along with an overall improvement in a feeling of wellbeing, are usually the first changes noticed. Next is a change in measurement, and drop in inches on the body. Often, the change in inches is seen in a "top down" fashion, meaning that inches will decrease in the neck, upper arms and chest region before decreasing in the midsection, abdomen, hips and thighs. Women are often most critical of this area of their body (the midsection), and it will appear to take the longest to see any results in the stomach. As you look down at the stomach it may not appear to be different, even though there are many changes occurring in the body.

After the inches start to go down, weight on the scale may begin to change. A healthy change in weight is anywhere from a half-pound to a pound per week. Any faster (although desirable to have a quick change) can be stressful on the body, resulting in a plateau, or rebound of weight. The slow and steady change in the body results in lasting change.

Emotionally, it can be tough to wait for this change to come around, but setting a future date with realistic goals is helpful. Example—a goal of two months later, dropping six to eight pounds. That is a success.

Chapter 15

Visceral Fat and Inflammation

Visceral fat is the fat that is in the abdomen, around the internal organs. This type of fat is noted for having the greatest impact on serious health conditions (heart disease, diabetes, stroke) but also stores the toxins and excess hormones within the body. Larger amounts of visceral fat also contribute to more inflammation in the body, causing plateaus and preventing weight loss. Without taking care of the inflammation, full results cannot be attained. Some tips to decrease inflammation include: cut out preservatives as much as possible, increase greens, increase antioxidants, cut sugar, add in vitamin D.

Chapter 16

Sleep

Menopause and the shift in hormones often brings a huge change in sleep. It can be difficult to get to sleep—and stay asleep. Sleep can be disrupted due to hot flashes. As the body metabolizes hormones at night, a surge (often progesterone) causes hot flashes, and then will disrupt sleep. The adrenaline that follows the hot flash is what will keep women awake at night.

Routines for Sleep

Sleep routines help your body get used to a pattern, allowing you to more easily fall and stay asleep. It's necessary to set aside time to begin a routine, which may be different than before. Often, women who can fall asleep quickly don't set enough time in their day for a good routine. Give yourself enough time to get the routine going. Routines include initiatives like going to sleep at the same time each night. Start with at least 30 minutes to get all these things done. Dimming lights and stopping activities on screen, using blue light-blocking glasses, diffusing soothing essential oils (lavender), reading or journaling are all calming activities to help wind down. The stress from the day can have a different impact than before, so it may take more time or added tactics in your routine to feel like your body is ready for sleep. This sleep process is necessary for hormonal health and repair of cellular tissue. We all know that if you get a bad night sleep, the next can be tough—difficult to wake and feel energized.

Adding in supplements can help with the sleep process: melatonin, chamomile, valerian, l-theonine, or others. Supplements should be used as an aid, but not as the only things to help with sleep. The overall routine is most important. Regular sleep can really change your body's ability to recover and rejuvenate, leading to a big shift in results.

Keeping some regularity in your schedule can also help with sleep. Having a set routine for going to bed and waking, along with consistent nutrition patterns, can help improve overall body function, including digestion. Setting a specific routine for workouts can help ensure they're worked into your schedule and getting done.

Routines can be tough for some women, but I promise you, schedules that provide more regularity will improve your health and make healthy things become habit.

Chapter 17

Stress and Cortisol

Stress is one of the most damaging things to the female body, and the most common thing for us to ignore. The changes that occur in perimenopause and menopause cause the body to process and metabolize hormones and other substances differently, and more slowly. Even the same amount of cortisol present (being under the same amount of stress as you have been over the past few years) can cause the body to be more overwhelmed with processing the stress.

I am going to refer to this as an increase in stress, even if the stress is the same amount, because it will seem like more stress to the body. If there actually is an increase in stress—any type of stress including emotional, physical, toxins (thoughts, trauma, toxins are the three categories of stressors)—this increase is even tougher to process and metabolize. This creates more inflammation in the body, contributing to increases in weight, pain, brain fog and more.

It's helpful to have a different expectation of stress on your new body. It will take a bit longer to work through, and you will have to do more to keep up with and process the amount of stress. Often, women don't realize that with a new body, they need to implement new daily routines to keep up with the processing of it all. It's not a bad thing, but just something to keep up with. I compare it to when you have longer hair, you have to brush it more often, or if you have a potential cavity, you must brush and floss more regularly to keep it from developing.

Any increase in stress can increase weight, slow the weight loss response or even result in weight gain. Many times, it can help to decrease stress if you are stuck at a plateau in results. Stress can be decreased by meditating, massage, chiropractic adjustments, acupuncture, adaptogens and more.

Chapter 18
Getting Back on Track: You Fell Off the Wagon, Now What?

It's human nature to fall off track with your goal, or feel like life circumstances have you taking two steps backward instead of forward. The most important thing is to keep the big picture in mind. View your progress in larger chunks of time. Rather than feeling bad that you didn't make it to the gym for a week, look at how many times you went over the past two or three months. Yes, daily habits are important when building consistency and have overall forward movement, but really looking at bigger chunks of time is what is going to help you make overall progress.

It can be easy to see a small set back as a much larger problem, and continue on the downward spiral. Have you ever had one piece of cake and thought "Well, I screwed everything up now, I may as well have two more pieces, a slice of pizza, an entire bottle of wine, and donuts for breakfast." Maybe not that dramatic, but you catch my drift.

My best advice is to allow yourself some wiggle room. Life is going to happen. If you are setting the expectation that you are going to be 100% strict and perfect on something, you are setting yourself up for failure. For the women I work with, I like to shift their thinking to not only teaching their body how to burn what they're eating, but as a lifestyle change. If you love chocolate, I'd rather have you allow yourself a piece or two when you want it, rather than binging on an entire bar on the weekend because you restricted yourself all week. When your body is healthy and functioning properly, it should have no problem burning those foods.

So if you do find yourself falling off the wagon, first ask yourself if the program you are trying to follow is too strict, or unrealistic for your life. If it is, it's time to find something that fits your lifestyle more seamlessly. If you don't think you are going to be able to keep it up forever, there's really no sense in starting only to set yourself up for failure. And hey, if you do "fall off the wagon," that's okay. Build it into your life, and jump right back on.

Chapter 19

Value of Herbs and Supplements to Your Overall Health

Adding in herbs and supplements does not take the place of a well-rounded, solid foundation of whole food nutrition. Supplements are meant to fill in the gaps, and herbs can take your results to the next level and be the linchpin when things hit the fan. The core five supplements and herbs to check out are multivitamin, fish oil, vitamin D, probiotics and adaptogens.

Supplements for menopause are key. With the above listed, be sure to get enough minerals daily—this can be done through mineral-rich protein shakes and other beverages including nuun, electrolyes, etc., but be sure these products are clean and do not contain any artificial colors or sweeteners). Most supplements for menopause are geared toward getting your body "back" like it was before menopause (estrogen-like supplements) but why not embrace the new phase of life you are in? In my opinion, supplements to mask symptoms are just a Band-Aid. If you want a true solution, you have to address the true problem.

If you are having symptoms, help your liver metabolize the excess hormones so it can regulate, allowing you to settle into the new phase of life that you are in. Things like black cohash are really popular but are only helpful for hot flashes, so if you don't have hot flashes and are really fatigued, it's not helpful.

These recommendations are blanket and general, and my specific recommendations per person depend on individual needs. Ultimately, if you are taking a supplement of some kind, it should have a positive impact on your health. If you are taking something and not noticing any differences, then it may not be getting fully absorbed, processed and metabolized. Check the quality of the supplements and any digestive issues to improve this.

Chapter 20

Hormone Replacement

Wtat do I need to know about it? There are a couple of different types of Hormone replacement therapy (HRT): regular HRT and BHRT (bioidentical HRT). Both add hormones to your system in an attempt to reinstate the hormonal effects of the body. The goal is to help with the negative symptoms that are associated with going through menopause.

Why is it being recommended to me? This is the one-track recommendation from some health professionals. There are limited tools that some medical professionals have in their tool bag, and this is the one they use.

Is there a better way? Many women have positive results when using their nutrition and supplements to help with the negative symptoms, but of course, you should reach out to a trusted health professional to help guide you through what may be the best options for you.

Part 6

In Conclusion...

We have been conditioned for far too long to accept that menopause is something we are just supposed to struggle through, while creams and supplements are thrown at us without any real information about why we're experiencing these symptoms.

Not anymore. You can start implementing the information provided in this book to take back control of your body and your health. Use this book as your compass to guide you through this phase of life, so you are no longer trying to survive menopause— instead, you will *thrive.*

If you are looking for more support or guidance individual to you, I encourage you to visit to my website at www.drbethwestie.com/programs and check out the 12-Week Menopause Program, where I put together all of the pieces for you, and help you customize the information to fit *you.*

Praise from those who successfully used Dr. Westie's program

" I was so stuck and frustrated, thinking I was going to have to live the rest of my life feeling that way. When I found Dr. Beth, I thought it was almost too good to be true. She was the only person speaking about menopause. I am so glad I trusted her and took the leap. I have tried every diet out there, and NOTHING provided the results this program has. I lost eight pounds, and 10 inches! I have more energy, and I finally feel like I have regained control of my body." – Cheryl T

"I tried everything that I used to do to lose weight, and nothing was working. I cut calories, added an extra workout, cleaned up my diet, and nothing. I was so lost, and couldn't stand the tire around my midsection anymore. I am so grateful to have found Dr. Beth. This is so much more than a weight loss program. I feel like I have control again, and know what to do to keep things on track. My hot flashes are gone, I'm sleeping better, no more mood swings, and I feel great. It's like I lost 10 years along with the 10 pounds. I couldn't be happier, I only wish I would have found her sooner!" – Jennifer T.

"I had tried EVERYTHING. You name it, I've done it. When talking with Dr. Beth, I quickly realized I had never taken my hormone issues into consideration. Having something custom to my body was clearly the answer. I'm down 25 inches, have my energy back, don't need an afternoon nap, and FINALLY feel like myself again." –Helen F.

"This might sound dramatic, but this program changed my life. I was feeling hopeless, lost, and completely out of touch with my body. Going through Menopause had been a terrible experience for me, and I couldn't find answers anywhere.
I was hesitant and skeptical that this would really work, but Dr. Beth was the only person that was talking about things specifically for Menopause. I am so glad I took a chance. I can't even explain my gratitude for Dr. Beth. I felt supported, and I know she truly cared about me. I have my life back. My energy has returned and I can do the things I love! I am down a couple pant sizes, but I actually feel in control again. This is priceless to me. I would do this again a million times over!" - Sandy J.

"My weight had been a struggle of mine for my entire life, or as long as I can remember. I had basically yo-yo dieted for my entire life. Jumping from one thing to the next hoping it was going to be the answer. As I got older it seemed like it got harder and harder to lose the weight. When I hit menopause it seemed like things spun out of control. When I started working with Dr. Beth it was so refreshing to find someone that looked at me as a whole. We talked *about my hormone issues, autoimmune issues, and my struggles with weight loss. She set up a plan specifically for me to address all of these things at once. It was life changing. The best investment I've made in my health. I had no idea I could feel this good. I am confident the tools I have been given have set me up for the rest of my life. My menopause symptoms are gone, auto immune issues under control, I'm down 27lbs and 30 inches overall. I feel like I have my life back. " Mary N.*

"Menopause hit me like a ton of bricks. Hot flashes, night sweats, insomnia, weight gain, you name it, I had it. It seemed like anywhere I turned there were only Band-Aids to put over these things, and not a real fix. I tried hormone replacement and that seemed like it made things worse. I tried to dig in and research, asked friends, doctors, my mom, no one had a real answer for me except "This is just part of this phase of life." In finding Dr. Beth it was like finally someone was speaking my language. I knew I didn't want to struggle through this, and she was the only real person that gave me hope. I joined her program and was astonished. There was so much I didn't know about my body it was almost embarrassing. Learning that my body was still having a hormone cycle even after a hysterectomy blew my mind. But when I started adding cooling and warming foods is was like my body thanked me for finally doing something right. My symptoms started to subside, I felt better, my energy was back, it was incredible. The things I learned in this program will serve me for the rest of my life. I've told every woman

I know about Dr. Beth because I truly feel she saved me from years of struggle and frustration." - Lisa S.

"Hi! I just wanted to stop by and let you know that at my gym they tested body fat along with weight and measurements before this challenge. And I know you say the scale isn't a good indicator of success, so I know you would like this. I am down 6% body fat since starting this program with you! I feel so much better, my clothes fit better, and I finally have the energy I was looking for! You have taught me so much about my body! THANK YOU!" – Abigail J.

"I had been going about weight loss in menopause all wrong. Who knew? Nothing that used to work was working, so I joined Dr. Beth's program. When she explained to me how important it was to detox excess hormone, and get my body metabolizing hormone again it made so much sense. I was trying to start at step 3 and had missed the first two steps. This program saved me so much frustration, money, headaches, time! I am so grateful for Dr. Beth. I feel like I finally have my life back. My energy is back, my weight is down, and I finally know how to eat for my body without dieting! I didn't think this was possible!" – Linda H.

"It's been over a year since I completed Dr. Beth's program and I am elated. I kept waiting for the other shoe to drop, but it hasn't and I know it won't. I've maintained my nutrition, energy, weight is still down. I am just so happy. I truly didn't think anything would ever really work for me long term. This is the real deal. If you never want to worry about your weight or have to diet again, you want to work with Dr. Beth! She is the best!" Jessica M.

"This is the real deal! Dr. Beth's passion for helping women learn how to feed their bodies and sustain their results is like nothing else. She has built something that is changing women's lives, mine included. I thought I would be dieting for the rest of my life, not anymore. I know what my body needs and when, and I've maintained my results for over 6 months now. I am in control, and I feel amazing. Words cannot describe how grateful I am!" – Tess N.

Resources

If you are ready to implement the information in this book in a way that is custom-design to fit your body, you're going to want to get on the waitlist for the next 12 Week Program at www.drbestwestie.com/waitlist, where you will get a behind-the-scenes look at what the 12 Week Program entails, and be the first to know when the next group starts! Join the waitlist at www.drbethwestie.com/waitlist.

If you don't want to wait for the next group program to open, and want to work together in a one-to-one capacity, you'll want to fill out the application at http://bit.ly/DrBethVIP and we will contact you to schedule your FREE one-to-one call with our team to help you determine which program is the right fit, and get you started.

Podcast: The Female Health Solution Podcast
YouTube: www.youtube.com/c/drbethwestie
Facebook: www.facebook.com/drbethwestie
Instagram: www.instagram.com/drbethwestie
Website: www.drbethwestie.com

REFERENCES

Westie, Beth. (2017). *The Female Fat Solution.* Minneapolis, Minnesota: BBI International.

Sims, Stacy, (2016). *ROAR.* City, State: Rodale Books.

Arciero, Paul. (2019). *The Protein Pacing Diet.* City, State: Outskirts Press.

Northrup, Christine. (2012 Revised). *The Wisdom of Menopause.* City, State: Bantam.

Winston, David, and Maines, Steve. (2007). *Adaptogens: Herbs for Strength, Stamina, and Stress Relief.* City, State: Inner Traditions/Bear & Company.

https://www.webmd.com/menopause/guide/menopause-hot-flashes

https://www.webmd.com/men/features/7-muscle-building-strategies-for-guys

https://www.livescience.com/63324-men-women-weight-loss-difference.html

https://www.menopause.org/for-women/menopauseflashes/mental-health-at-menopause/stress-getting-serious-about-solutions

https://www.healthline.com/nutrition/animal-vs-plant-protein#section1

https://www.isagenixhealth.net/tag/beet-juice/